ELE THERAPIES FOR PAIN RELIEF

THE IMPORTANCE OF PH BALANCE

CRIS ANGEL, DA, EAMP, HDD

outskirts press
DENVER, COLORADO

Electro Therapies for Pain Relief
The Importance of pH Balance
All Rights Reserved.
Copyright © 2014 Cris Angel, DA, EAMP, HDD
v1.0

Outskirts Press, Inc.
http://www.outskirtspress.com

ISBN: 978-1-4787-2865-8

Outskirts Press and the "OP" logo are trademarks belonging to Outskirts Press, Inc.

PRINTED IN THE UNITED STATES OF AMERICA

Table of Contents

Live A Happier, Longer Life: The Importance of pH Balance

Get the knowledge you need; k**nowledge on how to use solid proven scientific principles to live a happier and longer natural life**. Make more money and have more fun while you're on your way to peak performance; all while living life to your fullest potential by maintaining your body's proper pH Balance. Gain important information you need to know in this astonishing, well researched, but simple-to-read book. **You owe it to yourself and to those you love. Learn how to Live A Happier, Longer Life: The Importance of pH Balance.**

Disclaimer

The contents of this book are for consumer educational purposes only. Nothing contained in this book is or should be considered, or used as a substitute for professional medical advice, diagnosis or treatment.

The services provided in this book are to educate consumers on the ability of the body to maintain healing and optimal performance when pH Balance maintains between 6.8 and 7.5. This book and any suggestions in this book do not constitute the practice of any medical, nursing or other professional health care advice, diagnosis or treatment.

We advise users to always seek the advice of a physician or other qualified healthcare provider with any questions regarding personal health or medical conditions, be they mental, physical or emotional.

Never disregard, avoid or delay in obtaining medical advice from your doctor or other qualified healthcare provider because of something you have read in this book.

Introduction

Have you ever heard of machines ruling the world, using human beings as their energy source, by harvesting their bioelectrical energy and body heat?

A great sci-fi is the result of starting with a solid base of proven scientific principles, juiced-up by the freakiest possible consequences. And a great sci-non-fi is what makes you qualified to take control of proven scientific facts.

What you are going to gain from reading this extraordinarily researched, but simple-to-read book is the knowledge on how to use solid proven scientific principles, hence forward termed *scientific reality*, to live a happier and longer natural life while making more money and having more fun than you ever thought possible. All while you're living life to your fullest potential.

In writing this book, we'll attempt to keep it light, dash in a little humor now-and-again to make some of the technical information a bit more palatable. All the while, excuse the pun, to make sure your absorption level of the entire information presented gets fully optimized. In hopes of delivering valuable information to you about the ongoing important pH balance your body needs every second of every day. Your body is a work of art. Your body was designed by nature to be a perfect bioelectric machine.

CHAPTER 1

The Human Body: Your Perfect Bioelectric Machine

What? Never thought of your body as the *perfect bioelectric machine*? Perhaps your spouse or significant other can help you determine where you fall on a 1-10 scale of the PBM (perfect bioelectric machine).

All kidding aside, think again, you are the sum total of every single bite you put in your mouth. You are the sum total of every breath you breathe. You are a byproduct of your environment. It really is not as complicated as you might think.

History of Gastroenterology

No information in this book would be complete without knowing when gastroenterology was first discovered as a contributing factor in the overall functioning of the human body. An entire field of science opened up the morning of 6 June 1822.

Dr. William Beaumont came upon a severely wounded soldier. The soldier's wound was so serious it left his stomach permanently exposed through his abdominal wall. Dr. Beaumont performed a series of experiments and noted the presence of *hydrochloric acid* in the gastric juice. He immediately established the close working relationship between the emotional state and gastric secretion and digestion; noted the details of gastric motor activity and in his small way opened the gateway of physiological research and gastroenterology.

Stripped down to cell level, the human body is a network of micro generators and micro machines, dealing in Milli-volts and Nano-teslas.

Now, I might have lost you a bit, but stay with me on one of the most amazing journeys since the invention of *Carter's Little Liver Pills*.

Still lost? Well, Samuel J. Carter invented *Carter's Little Liver Pills* in Pennsylvania in the USA. The medicine had nothing to do with the liver, but was actually used to relieve back pain. I have no idea why Carter even used the word *liver* in the product's description –maybe he had beef liver for dinner the night he invented the pill.

I mention the relationship between what a thing is called and what it actually does based on performance, because you may believe two different things when you see a relationship without knowing all the facts. Carter invented pills to relieve back pain, then why call the pain reliever *Liver Pills*? As you may have guessed, one has nothing to do with the other.

In later years, the powers that be ordered the word "Liver" be taken from the product's name, but that fact is ancient history. We're here to discuss the ongoing important relationship you have with your body's pH balance.

Above point being, until you understand cell level performance, your body and its network of micro generators, you cannot possibly grasp how important it is to know how your amazing micro machine works in *promoting optimal healing and peak performance.*

For those who are familiar with the functions of the cells, electromagnetic force, and how the neural network operates in a human body, it is suggested that they go straight to the second chapter. However, if some memory refreshment is needed with cells in that area, it is worth the time spent on this first chapter.

Before touching on the term *Bioelectric machine*, let us learn about the cells, the neuron network, the way you feel *pain*, and how these variables actually work together.

The Human Body is Made of Cells

The human body is made of cells. The *cell* is the tiniest fragment of any living being, and it exists as an individual bio-machine. As a group, the cells make up the organs and other parts of your body.

You are a living, breathing, functioning product of the cells making up the essence of who you are daily. There are about 10 trillion cells divided into about 200 different types inside the average human body.

The Importance of Cells in Your Body

Why are the cells of your body so important? They are important, because:

- The cell is a structure that contains your DNA
- The cell contains enzymes
- The cell contains membranes
- The cell contains Proteins
- The cell contains chains of amino acids
- The cell is responsible for preventing infections
- The cell is responsible for reproduction
- The cell is responsible for repairing broken bones
- The cell is responsible for mending torn ligaments and muscles
- Much, much more…

All the tasks above, and more, occur at the cell level within your body.

DNA Instructs the Cells

The DNA tells the cell what to do. The enzymes present inside the cell are like busy workers on a mission, the cells:

- Break down the glucose

- Produce energy

- Build the cell walls

- Construct new enzymes

- Allow the cell to reproduce

- Cells use the amino acids as building blocks to build enzymes

- Cells use the amino acids as structural proteins

- Cells cause the necessary chemical reactions within your body to achieve all body functions

The Enzymes and Their Jobs

It is good to know about the enzymes and their jobs. For instance, some enzymes break the atoms and molecules of some chemicals, and others put them together. There more than a thousand types of enzymes, and there are specific enzymes that act as an efficient catalyst for a specific chemical reaction, speeding up that reaction tremendously.

Note: an example is always better for understanding the relationship between the cell and its driving force within the human body.

Let us take a look at the sugar *Maltose*. This sugar is made from two glucose molecules bonded together. The body needs individual molecules at the cell level. Enter the enzyme Maltase, as it breaks the bond and frees two glucose pieces.

If you or someone you know is diagnosed as being *Lactose intolerant*, you are probably familiar with the discomfort and limitations placed on those who suffer from *Lactose Intolerance*? Do you know why some of us can drink milk, enjoy milk products and the foods made with milk additives and others of us cannot?

Lactose is a type of sugar present in milk and present in products using milk as one of its ingredients. For instance, milk used in baked custards, cakes, ice-cream, dairy cream added to yummy mashed potatoes, right down to a delicious macaroni-n-cheese casserole, and lots more.

To digest milk, everything, including the sugar maltose, must be broken down into its glucose components. Lactase is the enzyme that is required here, and the intestinal cells of lactose-intolerant people do not produce this enzyme.

The above example shows the importance of enzymes, and the important role these cells play in producing the enzyme whenever they are needed.

Understanding the Neural Network

Let us get a fuller understanding of this neural network. What does a neural network do? Let's use our own nervous system, and see how it works.

Most of the sufferings of the body come in at the time in our lives when we should be feeling our fittest, old age, and most of the pain develops because the nervous system goes haywire. We shall read about the disorders of the nervous system in the next chapter. But for now, let us get a better understanding of how the nervous system works.

How the Nervous System Works

What is the nervous system? This is, again, a structure made of cells. Cells are named after the place or the organ where they populate. The cells in the nervous system are called *nerve cells* or *neuron cells*, and the structure looks like bundles of hairbreadth fiber optic cables; connecting the whole length and breadth of the body.

Nerve cells act like tinny busy-bodies who are constantly monitoring the intricate connectivity of every function of the body. From the pain you feel in the arch of your right foot, to the itch you feel behind your left ear, to the painful cavity in your upper molar that won't stop hurting.

The nerve cells constantly carry and deliver information through their collective superhighway of nerve fibers, often communicating in fractions of milliseconds to constantly monitor your entire body 24/7. Nerve cells form a network of pathways that consistently send out signals to keep you aware of pain, whether your pain is constant or increasing, or diminishing, makes you aware of pressure changes, atmospheric and internal, changes in temperatures, like hot, cold, clammy, etc.

Your amazing superhighway forms an intricate network that is continuously passing information along its amazing system of complex supercharged fibers.

Suppose a guy buys a liver transplant and forgets to pay. When he sees the Repo-man, he turns and runs. What happened here and why?

Though it is a complex thing that happens inside the network of neural fibers, let us try to make it simpler to figure out what happened to the guy that practices a spoof of grab-n-go, or consents to *this-for-that*, and then reneges.

Inside our brain and spinal cord, we have the *Association neurons* that decide on the action necessary to produce an end result. *Receptors*, the special neurons located in the ears and eyes of the person above who received the liver transplant, sees and hears the Repo man, and the *receptors or messengers* translate those sensory messages into nerve messages. These nerve messages are called *Nerve Impulses*. These *nerve impulses* travel along the *nerve fibers* at a high speed of up to 300 feet per second, through what are called *sensory neurons*. The sensory neurons carry the information from r*eceptors* in the *sense organs* to the *association neurons*.

After receiving the impulses, the association neurons analyze and interpret them. For instance, you are running across your kitchen floor bare footed and you suddenly step on a nail. It takes a fraction of a second for your brain to register the information sent via the sensory neurons.

By the time you go limping and screaming across the floor, the sensory neurons have already decided on the action you should take to distance yourself from the protruding sharp steel object on the floor. The message: get off the nail, buddy, run, flee the area posthaste.

These messages and messages like them are carried through the *motor neurons* and they reach the *Effectors* in the muscles and glands. As a result, you turn and run, and your heart pumps faster, followed by a few of your favorite well chosen words associated with sudden pain.

Receptors are available at the nerve ends, and they are situated all over our sensory organs. The sense of *Pain* or *Pleasure* is carried the same way, to the association neurons at the command centers situated within the spinal cord and brain.

On this note, one of the simplest and fastest ways for your physician or medical professional to determine spinal injury and to what extent of injury is to take a needle and prick the bottom of your toes, or stick various places on the bottom of your feet with a pin. A flinch on your part denotes feeling and a connection to the nerves in your spine. However, a lack of a response denotes a disconnect along the nerve fibers located in your spine.

The way the neurons carry the information is quite interesting.

The nerve impulses are nothing but electrical charges! It is plain old electricity flowing through the corresponding nerves, but at levels that could be called the tiniest of the tiny. The membranes of the nerve cells create electrical charges. Though there are many theories about what actually controls the production of each electrical charge, we shall discuss the much-accepted theory of cell membranes controlling it.

Theory of Cell Membranes

The membranes of the cells have pores that allow only certain substances to pass through. Diverse concentrations of some specific *ions* inside these cells and in their surrounding fluids create a potential electrical charge, by using certain electrochemical processes. As they control what goes inside or outside, the membranes play a vital part in the production of these electrical charges.

It is quite interesting to know how this *Electric Impulse* is created.

It is an important item as well, as we go onto the next chapters of utilizing the bioelectricity created inside our body. Let us see exactly what happens at the beginning of an Impulse. We have seen there are various chemical molecules present inside the cells and in the surrounding fluid. We have *Ions of Sodium*, *Potassium*, and also several organic ions in the mix. These are the basic things needed for the creation of electricity at the cellular level.

We also know the nerve cell membranes have special pores on them. The membranes too have some special *protein molecules*; which control their pores opening and closing. We also know that electricity is created when ions of different polarity, negative and positive ions, meet.

When the cells are at *Electrical Rest*, this is when they do not produce any impulses. There is still a voltage difference that exists across the membranes, between the insides and the outsides of the cells. This is referred to as the *Resting Potential*.

At this stage, the membrane keeps a low concentration of sodium ions inside, and at the same time maintains a higher concentration of potassium ions and negative organic ions in the surrounding fluids. These differences in the ion concentration make the inside of the nerve cell more negative than the outside, and hence the cell is *polarized*.

Before we go any further, let us examine the relationship between Polarization and Depolarization.

In simple terms, if the insides of a cell are more negative than the outsides, it is called *Polarization* of the cells. The reverse of this is called *Depolarization*.

No electricity is produced at this stage. We say the cells lay dormant (with all the potential to show up). What the cells need at this juncture is some sort of stimulus to depolarize them. When the cells are depolarized, the cells become positively charged and each cell fires. This firing is the basics for specific nerve impulses.

We have seen what is called: *the resting potential in a cell*. We know now if a stimulus is present, be it of a chemical, electrical, or mechanical nature, and this stimulus is applied to it, individual cells will change the structure of their pores, thereby affecting the travel of ions across the membranes.

When there is a stimulus, the sodium ions are allowed to be increased in the insides of individual cells, and this increase makes the insides of the cells positively charged.

In other words, *depolarization* takes place. The resting potential is changed, and if there is enough intensity, a certain threshold voltage occurs, and the cell becomes positively charged. As the cell becomes positively charged it fires. Each cell one-by-by communicates with the other instantly.

To give you another example of the speed at which this process occurs, take for instance, you are walking across a carpet made of nylon fibers. The friction between your body and the nylon fibers create a negative and positive connection and create a static electricity. You suddenly feel a sudden electrical shock or charge.

There is something unique about a neuron firing. When it fires, it fires away fully. There is no question of half firing or retarded firing or just leaking. Whatever might be the intensity of the stimulus, the neuron fires with full intent, and the impulses are all of the same size and time duration.

This uniqueness in the firing of the neurons is called rightly as the *all-or-nothing way of the neurons*. The vivid listener may raise their hand and ask how the brain could detect the intensity of a stimulus, if the size and duration are one and the same. That is a valid question.

The brain calculates the total number of nerve fibers stimulated, and the frequencies at which the impulses are generated, and decides on the strength of the impulse. For instance, you wouldn't flee your home if you received a static electrical shock as you walked across your living room carpet, but if you're standing in the middle of a field during a lightning storm and it's pouring down rain, your brain will quickly calculate through nerve fiber stimulation that you need to get to a safe, dry place to avoid being struck by lightning.

How does your body know you are in danger of being struck by lightning during an electrical storm? The clouds have positive and negative charges (+ -) and so do the nerve cells in your body. You must place yourself out of harm's way or play the game of Russian Roulette and hope you avoid injury or death.

Having learnt the basics in the electricity and impulse generation, let us learn some relatively tougher terms in the transmission of these impulses. Again, we are trying to make them sound simple, and once more we will continue to keep it simple in hope of advancing your understand of how your amazing body works.

Two Types of Protoplasmic Protrusions: Axons and Dendrites

Before we begin this section you should know what these terms mean:

- Axon

- Myelinated Axon

- The Nodes of Ranvier

- Synapses

- Neurotransmitters

- Postsynaptic Potential

Do not let the words scare you, as some folks may decide the words sound like the names and words from the next installment of the famous serial *Harry Inside the Matrix*. Let us meet the awesome six and see what all the fuss is about.

The Awesome Six Terms & Their Functions

Axons and *Dendrites* are the two types of proto-plasmic protrusions that extrude from the cell body of a neuron. They are different from each other by their shapes and lengths, and usually the Axon transmits, while the Dendrite receives a signal. We say *usually*, because some neuron types have no Axons and they transmit signals from their Dendrites. The Axon is slightly projected away from the cell body, the *Soma*. It is designed to safely conduct the electrical impulses away from the Soma. Axons are the primary transmission lines of the nervous system. They make up the nerves as they form together as bundles.

Myelinated Axon is the Axon with a sheath called *Myelin*, a dielectric, an electrically insulating material which forms a layer around the axon of a neuron called the *myelin sheath*. One can find the axons of many neurons sheathed in myelin, mostly in the bodies of vertebrates. Sheathing with myelin is called *Myelination*. Note: *Saltation,* a rapid mode of electrical impulse propagation, becomes possible with this Myelination.

Along the myelinated nerve fibers, there are gaps occurring at perfect intervals. These gaps lack the myelin sheath, and hence they are the unmyelinated segments of the axon. These are like Nodes, and are called the *Nodes of Ranvier.* These are the places where action potentials are amplified and transmitted down the axon.

Conduction along the Axon

As we are now familiar with the above terms, let us look at the Conduction along the *Axon*. A solution that is capable of conducting electric charges as a current is topped inside an Axon. Depolarization takes place. But, this depolarization in one area of the axon is then spread to the neighboring areas all along the axon in a wave-like pattern, through the topped up solution. This is called the *action potential*. The *myelin sheath* plays an important part here. The nerve impulses sweep continuously along the axon, but they can occur only at the *Nodes of Ranvier*. In case the axon has the myelin sheath. With the *myelin sheath*, the impulses actually travel, jumping from one node to another. There are, however, incidences when it has no myelin sheath.

So far, it is all quite interesting. Now, let us know what Synapses, Neurotransmitters, and Postsynaptic Potential, mean. And, let us maintain that interest in understanding these terms.

Synapses are functional connections that are made between neurons, or between neurons and other types of cells in the body, like the muscle cells or the organ cells. Synapses help regulate the constant flow of nerve impulses throughout the nervous system. Synapses can be of Electrical or Chemical types, the ways the connections are made between the neuron cells themselves, or between them and the other types of cells, to pass on the information.

When we further explain the passing of information between the cells, we would come across terms like *Presynaptic*, *Postsynaptic*, and *Synaptic Cleft*. What is Presynaptic and Postsynaptic?

When a connection is made, it could be 20–40 nm distant if it is chemical, and it could be 3–4 nm distant if it is electrical. The sending end is called as *Presynaptic* and the receiving end of that connection is called as *Postsynaptic*. The gap between the chatting cells is called as the *Synaptic Cleft*.

Neurotransmitters: Endogenous Chemicals

Neurotransmitters are a certain group of chemicals called the *Endogenous chemicals*, which transmit the signals when a synapse occurs. They are synthesized from precursors, like the amino acids obtained from the simple conversion of diet or otherwise. Neurotransmitters are enclosed in *Synaptic Vesicles*, small membrane-bound spheres, which are docked at the presynaptic plasma membrane. These regions are called *Active Zones*.

In the transmission of information across *Synapses*, when an impulse reaches the end of an axon, the neurotransmitters from the information-sending cell are released into the synaptic cleft, where they reach onto the receptors in the membrane of the information-receiving cell. There they truss-on to those receptors. Release of neurotransmitters usually follows after an Action potential develops at the synapse. But sometimes, graded electrical potentials do the initiation. And other times, Low-level releases, also referred to as Baseline *releases*, occur even without this electrical stimulation.

Let us go a bit deeper and see what happens when the neurotransmitters reach the next cell, in the neuron-to-neuron transmission. When they get to the dendrites of the next nerve cell they open up some pores of the nerve membrane. Postsynaptic Potential, a kind of voltage change, follows because some ions would move through these pores. Depending upon the action or inaction that follows, this postsynaptic potential can be either inhibitory or excitatory.

What is the difference? Not every impulse that reaches a synapse is transmitted to the next neuron. In an inhibitory postsynaptic potential, the axon is prevented from producing another action potential, whereas, an excitatory postsynaptic potential tends to produce another action potential as it spreads to the axon of that nerve cell.

Earlier, we saw that the firing of a neuron cell, in passing on information as an impulse, shall be its fullest. We have also seen that the brain calculates the strength of the impulse by the total number of nerve fibers stimulated, and we noted the frequencies at which those impulses are generated. Since the size and duration would be one and the same, it is worthwhile to learn further on this; for these actions involve modulation of amplitude and the role of the electricity in memory-related activities of the brain.

Presynaptic Action Potential

The brain defines the strength of a synapse by the amplitude of the change in membrane potential that happens as a result of a *presynaptic action potential*. In other words, the number and size of each of the connections from the message-sending neuron to the message-receiving neuron, enable the brain to calculate the strength of a synapse. Ask any teenager what a PSP is, but here, PSP denotes the Postsynaptic Potential. The amplitude of a PSP could measure between 0.35-0.4mV. That is a low one. On the higher side, it could be about 20mV.

It should be noted that these PSPs could be modulated. Here comes the Neuromodulators. What are they?

These are certain chemicals, like *dopamine*, *serotonin*, *acetylcholine*, and *histamine* that make one neuron use different neurotransmitters to connect to several neurons at once, as opposed to the direct synaptic transmission; in which one message-sending neuron directly influences the other message-receiving neuron. Though we are talking about chemicals, the idea is to understand how the amplitude of a PSP can be modulated as a result of a change in the previous activity.

LTP, the *Long-term Potentiation*, is the change in synaptic strength that can last long, maybe lasting hours. Likewise, these changes could be of short-term nature, STP, lasting a few seconds to a few minutes. A system, known as the s*ynaptic plasticity*, is associated with the learning and memory capabilities. This is a term, describing the long-term changes in synaptic strength.

The last few paragraphs were a bit on the hard side, no doubt, but they were equally interesting, right?

Having learned several important things, like, how the cells work, and how the neural system works, now it is easier to comprehend how a p*ain* is felt. This will sincerely help you master the *Pain Management Studies*, described in the later chapters of this book.

- What is pain and how do we feel it?
- What really happens inside the body, when a pain is experienced?

We have to see the neurobiology of pain to answer these questions. Many would explain it as *an unpleasant sensory and emotional experience.*

Well, it need not be unpleasant all the time. It all depends upon the mindset with which we face anything in life. But, since most of us would rather go to any extend to avoid this sensory experience; it is worth our time to know how it is felt, and what it is all about.

In the following few pages, we shall see what happens inside our body at the cellular level as we are experiencing pain. We shall also see its electrical nature, how it is transmitted and where, and we will look at the different types of pain.

If a single broad classification of a problem takes up most of the time for most of the people engaged in the medical field as professionals, it would surely be to address *pain* and all its implications.

That said; it is also hard to define. For pain is more of a subjective nature. It is what and where the sufferer says it is. However, we can be certain of one thing; pain is something one feels as a warning that something bad is causing or about to cause damage to the body, somewhere, somehow, and one should do something about stopping it.

Nociception is the word for the perception of *pain*, and there are several types of this Nociception. Generally, the stimulation is relayed to the CNS, the *central nervous system*, in four acts.

The first act is the *Stimulation*. The stimuli can be of a mechanical nature or of a chemical nature. Getting a burn, thermal or chemical, can be put in the later, while pressure, puncture, or a cut, can be put in the former.

The second act is the contact with the stimulus, the *Reception*. In reception, the nerve-end comes in contact with and senses the stimulus.

The third is the *Transmission*. This is where the nerve sends the signal to the central nervous system. Then the information is relayed, engaging several neurons within the CNS.

The fourth act is the *Pain-center Reception*. This is when the brain receives the information for further analysis and action.

Now, let us see how CNS receives the information as it is relayed from the site of stimulation.

We have already seen that receptors are fired by a group of neuron cells in a normal sensory perception, like the *Touch* and the *Temperature*, etc. These can be classified as *non-painful stimuli*, and receptors involved here are the *Somatic type*. But in *Nociception*, another type of neurons, called the *Nociceptors*, go into action first. Normally, Nociception uses different neural pathways than normal perception.

Let us see more about Act 4, the *Pain Signal Reception*.

The Nociceptors are found in any area of the body, either externally or internally that can sense pain. The skin, cornea, and mucosa are the external areas, and the muscles, joints, bladders, guts, and a variety of organs are the internal areas; where you can find them.

Inside the spine, there is the *dorsal root ganglia* of peripheral nerves and the Nociceptors' cell bodies lay therein. They are available in the *trigeminal ganglia* too. These ganglia of specialized nerves are for the face, while the dorsal root ganglia are for the rest of the body. The axons of these neurons terminate in branches to form receptive fields after extending into the peripheral nervous system.

The *Nociceptor neurons* travel in the *peripheral sensory nerves*, the same way normal sensory neurons do. But, the normal neurons are *myelin sheathed*, and conduct quickly at their special endings, with which they sense the feelings, like the Touch or Pressure, whereas, the Nociceptors conduct the sense of pain through their free nerve endings. Since they are not myelin sheathed their action is comparatively slower.

There are three classes of Nociceptors.

- First category, Pressure and Touch Stimulus Sensing *Mechanosensitive Receptors*. They are lightly myelinated and faster conducting. These are the A-fibers.

- Second category is the *Mechanothermal Receptors* that are lightly myelinated and faster conducting. They respond to mechanical stimuli like Pressure or Touch, as well as the thermal stimuli like Heat. These are the A-delta fibers. A-delta fibers are sensory fibers, conduct signals more rapidly than unmyelinated C- fibers, but more slowly than the first category A-fibers.

You can easily remember them, as they are the ones that make you withdraw your hand in a flash if you touch a hot Barbeque plate. The *Polymodal Nociceptors* that are the C-fibers belong to the third category. These are the unmyelinated and slowly conducting neurons that respond to a variety of stimuli.

Now that you know about the all-important Nociceptors in sensing pain, it is time to cut your little finger. Don't be alarmed! All we are trying to do is an imaginary performance, just assuming that a sharp object has accidentally cut a finger. Just imagine, don't do it for God sake, even if you completely agree with the motto of, *anything for Science.*

What happens when a finger is cut? There is this reception of pain. First, there is the mechanical stimulation from the sharp object. Then, Potassium ions are released from the insides of the damaged cells. Inflammation takes place, and *Prostaglandins*, *Histamines*, and *Bradykinin* from the immune cells that invade the area and Substance P from the nearby nerve fibers all accumulate there. These are the substances that cause the action potentials in the Nociceptor neurons.

You would feel pain, of course. If you notice carefully, there would be two types of pain. The first type of pain is of an intense kind. You feel it immediately the moment you cut your finger. The A-delta Nociceptors conduct this.

The second type of pain follows directly, but it will be rather slow, prolonged, and you'll experience a dull ache. The slower C-fibers Nociceptors conduct this.

At this juncture, we should know about the latest development. Either of the Nociceptors can be blocked and the two types of pains can be separated and controlled.

As you try not to jump up-and-down, holding your cut finger, let us see how the *Pain Signal* is transmitted.

The dorsal roots carry the signals from the cut straight away into the spinal cord.

Within the dorsal horn, the signals make the necessary synapses on the neurons. Synapses of the neurons occur within the spinal cord segment at the point of entry; as well as one to two segments above and below. In some injuries, like internal injuries, sometimes it becomes difficult to determine the exact location of the pain, because of this multiple connections. They might relate to a broader area of the body.

Now, we shall see what happens with a face injury, the Pain Signals from the face. You can leave the hand, and assume that you have cut yourself, just a nick though, right under your nose. Pun not intended.

The *Somatosensory neurons*, from the face and head, travel into the central nervous system through the nerve called the *Trigeminal nerve*. This is like having a mini spinal cord, especially for your face. The connection goes all the way to the brain, the mid-medulla and in the lower medulla regions. The signals synapse in the group of neurons there, and through the *tregeminal-thalamic tract* within the midbrain they reach the *thalamus*.

For those who don't know, the Thalamus is the part of our brain, sending out nerve fibers to relay sensation, spatial sense, and motor signals to the *cerebral cortex*, along with the regulation of consciousness, arousal, sleep, and alertness. This is situated between the cerebral cortex and midbrain.

It should be noted here, excluding the *olfactory system*, all other sensory systems include a *thalamic nucleus* that receives sensory signals and sends them to the associated primary *cortical area*. When the signals about the nick under the nose reach here, neurons in the thalamus take over and they further relay the signals onto the *Somatosensory cortex* and *Limbic system*.

The Somatosensory cortex is the area where the signals are registered, and the Limbic system supports a variety of functions including emotion, behavior, long-term memory, and olfaction. It is a set of brain structures that includes the *hippocampus, amygdala, anterior thalamic nuclei, septum, limbic cortex and fornix.*

Now, we have seen how Pain Signals are received from the face and the head side, and from the other parts of the body. Let us also investigate the *Spinothalamic tract.* The center of the spinal cord looks like a piece of thick spaghetti made up of white matter. This is called the Spinothalamic tract. If the injury is from the other areas of the body, the signals reach this tract, and then they travel up the spinal cord through the *brain stem* known as the *Medulla*, and synapse on neurons in the thalamus (the brain's relay center), which we have already seen. The nerve fibers from the thalamus then relay the signal to various areas of the somatosensory cortex.

Pathways of Pain

Having understood the Pain Signals and how they travel, it is now time to go a little deeper and see about the *Pathways of Pain*. This is not to be confused with how they travel. We are trying to understand the different types of pain and the various routes they take so that we can further decide on the better applications in managing them.

First, let us see the types of Pain. *Acute Pain* is the pain that comes after an injury to the body. It is a message that warns about potential damage and requests an action from the brain. This could be either slow or quick, and could last for about six months on the longer side, or just a few minutes on the shorter side. This type of pain goes away as the injury heals.

Chronic pain is another type of pain that persists long after the injury is gone. Sometimes, in the absence of any injury too, this pain would persist. Lasting for periods of more than six months, this pain usually does not request the body to respond. The pain asso-ciated with malignant tumors, invasive procedures, or treatments of such nature, is called as *Cancer pain*. The pressure on the nerves, exerted by the invasion of the tumor onto the healthy tissues, and also by the injured cells by the invasive procedures, causes the pain.

As of today, scientists are still carrying out research on ways to find out how exactly the pain information is processed inside the brain. So far, we know that once the signals reach the motor cortex, they travel further through the spinal cord to reach the motor nerves to draw an action. The action is caused by the muscle contractions, triggered by the impulses. That is why if the injury happens on the hand, immediately you pull away your hand.

But the brain is capable of influencing the percep-tion of pain. You might have noticed, every time after an injury the intensity of the pain gets less and less and eventually goes away. Sometimes, if one consciously gets distracted, either through the external efforts or just on one's own, there will be less of pain. And, we all know about the use of placebos, dummy tablets that suggest that they are painkillers.

Note: These are all possible only because the pain-influencing neural pathways originate in the so-matosensory cortex, which relays the signals to the thalamus, and then onto the hypothalamus. The neurons from the thalamus descend to the midbrain, and synapse on ascending pathways in the medulla and spinal cord. The ascending nerve signals, which are thus inhibited, produce the pain-relief in the form of stimulation of natural pain-relieving opiate neurotransmitters, like the *Endorphins, Dynorphins* and *Enkephalins*.

Physiological and psychological factors could influence the perception of pain. As the circuitry of the brain normally degenerates with age, older people have lower pain-enduring capacity, and hence have more problems about it. Young people too, regardless of age, when the body is stressed from lack of sleep, experience more pain.

The memory factor too plays a major role in influencing the neural responses, as the signals are processed in the *limbic system*, which is directly connected to the memory files. The sex-linked genetic traits and hormonal changes in women allows them posses a higher sensitivity to pain than men. For men, it could be a psychosocial factor, to endure more pain and not show it. This would make you wonder why the drug Morphine is named that way, other than what the word Morph suggests, *more pain*?

As we find out about the physiological and psychological factors that could influence the perception of pain, it is worth our time in learning another important theory connected with the emotional influence. This theory is called as the *Gate Control Theory of Pain.*

In the year 1965, Ronald Melzack and Patrick Wall opined that there should be a gating mechanism within the dorsal horn of the spinal cord, which allows the thoughts and emotions to influence the perception of pain. They explained that the small nerve fibers, the pain receptors, and large nerve fibers, the normal receptors, synapse on the Projection cells, and the signals go up the spinothalamic tract to the brain.

So, there will be two kinds of signaling. Signal One travels from the injured place to the inhibitory and transmission cells, and then onto the brain through the spinal cord. Signal number two travels directly up the cord to the brain, from the injured place. It bypasses the inhibitory and transmission cells. At the brain, a signal may be triggered back down the spinal cord to lessen the pain intensity, by modulating the inhibitory cell activity.

According to this theory, the spinal cord contains a *neurological gate*, which could allow or not allow the pain signals to continue on to the brain. This gate operates by differentiating between the thin and thick types of fibers carrying pain signals. While the thin fibers impede the inhibitory cells and leave the gate open, the thick fibers excite the inhibitory cells and close the gate. Thus, Pain signals traveling through the small nerve fibers are allowed to pass through, while those relayed by the large nerve fibers are blocked.

How can you use this theory? Next time someone bangs your finger with something heavy, rub it thoroughly, the place, not that heavy something. You would stimulate much of the normal somatosensory inputs to the projector neurons. The Gate is closed and the perception of pain is reduced.

This *Gate Control Theory* sometimes explains phantom pain and chronic pain effectively.

Hypnosis, Acupuncture, Massage Therapy, Biofeedback, Medications, Surgery, or a combination of two or more of these, are used to help the sufferers of pain, in the effective management of it.

In the coming chapters, we will be learning more on the usage of mild electricity in managing the pain. But, right now, we shall also see about the other methods and how they act.

Before we get into that, we must know that there is no absolute measurement of the degree of pain. For pain is a subjective matter. However, the medical professionals use the numerical rating scales, and ask their patients to identify their pain intensity on a pain-scale of 0-10. Sometimes, pictures of faces expressing vary-ing degrees of pain are also used.

Shall we see what happens when *aspirin, acetamin-ophen, ibuprofen,* and other non-opioid analgesics are used to reduce the pain?

First, the injury happens.

Second, the damaged tissues let loose a good amount of enzymes, stimulating the local pain receptors.

Third, the non-opioid analgesics interfere with the enzymes and reduce pain, as well as the inflammation.

Fourth, sometimes, with prolonged use, gastro-intestinal discomfort and bleeding occurs in the liver and/or kidneys.

What happens with the Opioid analgesics like, *morphine, meripidine, propoxyphene, fentanyl, oxyco-done* or *codeine?*

These Opioid analgesics bind on to the natural opioid receptors and act on the synaptic transmission in the central nervous system. They activate the de-scending pathways to lessen the pain and inhibit the ascending pathways for less pain perception. There is a good chance of reducing any higher levels of pain, but also there is a very good chance of overdosing, and becoming an addict.

Co-analgesics, also called as *Adjuvant analgesics*, are sometimes used for relieving chronic pain that comes from injury to the central nervous system, the Neuropathic pain. Though there main use is for something else, they still work. For example, the anti-epileptic drugs reduce the membrane excitability.

We know that by reducing the membrane excitability, the CNS neurons' action potential conduction is also reduced. If the pain-modulating pathways were affected, the synaptic transmission of *serotonin* and *norepinephrine neurons* in the CNS also gets affected.

The *Tricyclic antidepressants* act in the above said manner. Anesthetics like the lidocaine, novocaine and *benzocaine*, interfere with the sodium and potassium channels in the nerve cell membranes, and block their action potential transmission.

In other pain management practices, the chiropractor with his extensive knowledge of the neuro-musculoskeletal system manipulates the joints to relieve compression of the nerves.

Massage Therapy is another example of the Gate theory, as it stimulates blood flow and relieves muscle spasms. The increased somatosensory signals in turn relieve the pain. Cold applications reduce the inflammation, while hot applications increase the blood flow, both contributing to the lessening of pain.

In a particular method, tiny electrodes are used on the skin to stimulate it. In the *Acupuncture* method, nerve cells are stimulated to release *endorphins*. These are again the procedures attributed to the practical usage of the *Gate Theory*.

How Electricity is Involved in the Well-Being of Cells

Now, we come to the important section of this first chapter; how electricity is involved in the well-being of our cells.

How does our body make electricity, and how does our body make use of that electricity? Though we have seen how in the previous pages, let us read more.

We were going through the Cell membrane's capacity to control what goes in or out in the first few pages of this chapter. Many of us know the importance of the tiny voltages and currents that run inside the body, but many of us would like to know more on how it is produced and how it is used.

Previously, we learned about the Synapses. The Synapses, the Signals, the Heartbeats, all these occur, because of the electricity produced by our bodies. It was electricity traveling to convey messages from one point to another when we were talking about the firing of the synapses, the nervous system relaying impulses, the commands coming from the brain to withdraw your hand if you touch a hot barbeque plate.

In today's information superhighways, they say digital information is passed in Zeros and Ones. In the outside world, electricity passes through cables, and carries that information to its destination.

Inside our body, it is the *Cell* that fires or does not fire, and it is the cell that produces the information to be relayed through nerve fibers and the neural system to various parts of the body.

Instead of traveling, the signal is flashed, picked up, flashed again by the cells through their synapses. The message reaches its destination in this relayed fashion.

An important signaling system inside our body, relayed by electricity as explained above is relayed through our *Pulse*. The *Sinoatrial node*, or SA node, located in the right Atrium of our heart controls the rhythm of our heartbeat and the movement of blood from the heart to the other parts of the body. Sensing danger and supplying more blood to the required parts is done this way.

What our senses find, what our various organs and body parts do, all these are communicated and commandeered by the electricity produced by the respective cells. All communications that happen are relayed by the right amount of electricity produced by the cells.

Let us look again into the way this electricity is produced by our cells.

All the cells in our body are charged either positively or negatively. Those that are not sending any message are negatively charged, and those that are actively sending a message are positively charged at the respective moments.

We know that Potassium ions are negative, and *Sodium ions* are positive. In the normal stage, the cells have more ions of Potassium, and less ions of Sodium than the fluid outside. The outside fluid has the reverse kind. Since Potassium ions mean negative, the cell at the resting stage can be called *slightly negative charged*. Since Sodium ions are positive, the surrounding fluid that is the outsides of the cell, having more of those ions can be called *slightly positive charged*. We must note that both areas are only slightly charged either way, and there would not be sufficient charge-difference to make electricity at that cell resting moment.

The membranes of the cells have the capacity to control what goes in or out. When prompted by the need to make a signal, the membrane allows the ions to go in or out freely, of course, *Free* as in a communist country in a controlled manner.

Sodium and Potassium ions move freely through the membrane, as the negative Potassium ions are attracted by the positive Sodium ions. So do the Sodium ions in the reverse. This is called the Sodium-Potassium Gate. This opens when a message needs to be relayed.

The flip between positive and negative charges can be called as the *Zeros and Ones Switch*. Through the acts of Synapses, the impulses created by the switch are carried from cell to cell, relayed until the destination is reached.

We have read about the SA node, previously. If that node misfires, if the right signal is not produced or relayed, it causes an extra heartbeat or one less heartbeat. Palpitation occurs. That is one of the minor problems, if you consider what happens to a sensitive electrical machine, as in when a power surge occurs. The whole body depends on the right amount of electricity produced by the cells for functioning and communicating.

In the case of an electrical shock, what happens is kind of akin to an electrical surge. Just imagine what would happen in case of a lightning striking the body. Engineers refer such mishaps as *All Circuits Fried-up*. But most of the times, our cells can repair themselves, and a fry-out need not be the end of matters. If the cells are made to produce the right amount of electricity at the right time the body should function as a smooth as a Rolls Royce.

If the proper amount of electricity were not produced, proper information would not be relayed properly. Well, this could be a dramatic statement with word play, but one word that describes the importance of electricity produced in the cells is *properly*.

Having understood the electrical nature of the body and the connection between the working of a Body Cell and Electricity, we shall now go to the effects of *Electro Magnetic Field*, EMF.

For those who do not know what an EMF is, it can be described as a *physical field produced by electrically charged objects*, and *it directly and indirectly affects the behavior of charged objects in the vicinity of that field*. It is one of the four fundamental forces of nature, like Gravitation, and extends indefinitely throughout Space.

Moreover, when viewed with proper equipment, it looks like a combination of an electric field and a magnetic field. The two sources of this field are, the *Electric field* produced by stationary charges, and the *Magnetic field* produced by the moving charges.

Note: Maxwell's Equations and the *Lorentz Force Law* are the rules that better describe the ways in which charges and currents interact with this EMF.

Understanding the EMF is important for it leads to the understanding of the next subject, the

Electromagnetic Radiation. The Electromagnetic Radiation is everywhere, and it affects the health of the body one way or other.

Before understanding the electromagnetic radiation health effects to the body, one must know how body cells function, and that is what we accomplished in the previous pages.

We have seen that there is subtle electrical activity similar to electric circuits in our body. These electrical currents can be equated with the flow of blood in terms of their important to the well-being of the body. Any untoward disturbance could lead to quite a bit of destruction to the effective functioning schedule of all organ systems, especially that of the brain. Growth, metabolism, thought and other vital bodily functions are controlled by this electrical activity and the disturbance might even lead to diseases, including the development of cancer.

We are all basically electromagnetic beings, with tiny electrical currents existing inside us because of chemical reactions in our cells. The digestive process and the activities of the brain, the pumping of heart, the resulting biochemical processes, all these are the result of the rearrangement of charged particles. Across arteries, veins, and capillary walls, electric currents flow through, and voltages generate and fluctuate. The electricity makes the white blood cells and metabolic compounds to slip through the walls of the tissues. By the transmission of electric impulses the nerves relay signals.

The foundation of the healing process in case of injuries is this electrical system. The balancing act in the processes of all internal organs is also due to the same electrical system. A sensitive electromagnetic system that runs on millivolts, the body is actually a bioelectric machine. Since it is like an electromagnetic machine, it has got its own Electromagnetic frequencies that act at various important places inside.

Note: Any exposure to external frequencies from the surrounding environment, however small they are, could have positive or negative effects on these internal systems.

The direct exposure to higher-than-normal electromagnetic fields could cause nerve, muscle, and hair stimulation. On the bad side, exposure to a particular external frequency consistently for more than a few minutes is sure to disrupt the body's ability to run its own electrical circuitry at optimum efficiency.

CHAPTER **2**

Your Body in Perfect pH Balance

A body in perfect balance is like a fine oiled and fine tuned working machine. Your body's pH balance is essential to your good health. Maintaining your body's proper pH balance is vital to your health in avoiding chronic and degenerative diseases. As you and I age, keeping and maintaining the acid/alkaline balance of our bodies is essential to our physical well-being.

The truth is your entire body was designed to be in perfect synchronization with all its working parts. Think of your surround sound system you may have on your television or synchronized with your other working devices in your entertainment center. When one wire is disconnected it affects the quality of the sound you hear. Your body is no different. When your body is out of synch you may feel the effects in your bones, joints, and you may feel it in the overall working functions within your body, from osteoporosis to weakness.

Your body was never created to be out of harmony with all its working parts. It was designed to be in harmonious interaction with every cell in your body. When your body is out of sync, out of pH balance, how can you expect to physically feel? You may suffer:

- A General Feeling of Malaise
- Bad Breath
- Burning Sensation on the Tongue
- Burning Sensations in the Mouth
- Diabetes
- Dry, Pungent Smelling, Firm Stools
- Fatigue
- Fibromyalgia
- Foul Smelling Runny Stools
- Frequent Colds
- Frequent Flu and Flu-Like Symptoms
- Frequent Sighing
- Heart Disease
- High Cholesterol Levels
- Inability to Think Straight
- Joint Pain

- Lack of Sleep
- Low Blood Pressure
- Muscle Aches
- Muscle Pain
- Rheumatoid Arthritis
- Sensitivity to Acidic Fruits and/or Vinegar
- Sores or Fleshy Projections on Top Your Tongue
- Sunken, Recessed Eyes
- Trouble Swallowing
- Unpleasant Smelling Perspiration
- Water retention
- Weakness

We know how it makes you feel, but how does one get their pH out of balance in the first place?

Three of the biggest culprits to disrupting your body's normal pH balance are food, drug use, and illness. We'll address the biggest offender first, legal medications.

Folks in the USA are notorious for taking large amounts of prescription drugs. A man once said he took twenty-seven different prescription drugs. When asked, "Why in the world would you take so many pills?" His explanation was telling of so many of us. He said, "Most of the medicine I take is to prevent the side effects of another medicine I take." What?

He went on to explain, "This medicine in this bottle is for the side effect of diarrhea this other medicine causes. This pill is for headache caused by this medicine. This medicine is for fluid retention caused by this medicine, etc. etc.

As he pointed at each one, I, frankly, admired his level of knowledge about each medication he took and its individual counter effect.

As he continued, he pointed at each medicine bottle in a small brown suitcase of sorts and explained the drug interaction of each one. When I asked him how many medicines he started taking when he first visited a doctor, I was shocked when he said, "Actually, I believe I may only need the first two prescribed to me. All the rest counteract side effects of others prescribed by my physician over a period of several years."

Then I asked him the million dollar question, "Why would you take dozens of medications to counteract two of your initial medications if you thought you didn't need to take them?"

His answer may shock you. "Well, I take them because Dr. Smith (not his real surname) is my doctor. He knows what's best for me."

When you look at the larger picture of the population, most of us quickly see the correlation between *deaths* and the *cause of death*. For instance, is it any wonder so many people die of *sclerosis of the liver* who have never drank alcoholic beverages or used illegal drugs? Is it any wonder large numbers of people die from *kidney failure*? The list goes on and on…

For most of the population as a whole, the ideal body pH balance is a bit more alkaline than it is acid. Throughout your day, your body is constantly regulating itself, attempting to balance the acid/alkaline in your body. One central player in regulating your body's pH balance is *calcium.*

Calcium is a mineral. In fact, it is one of the most prevalent and most abundant minerals in your body and is necessary for the proper working order of every cell in your body. To better understand the importance calcium plays in your body, think back on a blood test your doctor may have ordered for you.

When your doctor orders blood work, you go to a lab and a lab tech draws blood. Sometimes the tech may also request a urine sample from you to do a urinalysis. Then after the lab tech analyzes the results, they are forwarded to your doctor. Your doctor in turn studies the results, and he or she too analysis the results again. One of the numbers your doctor looks at when he studies your lab results is your *calcium level* number.

A good calcium level is within the range of 8.4 – 10.2, and should always be less than 10.0 mg/dl for those forty-years-old and over.

When calcium levels are low, your body will take calcium from your bones in an attempt to maintain sufficient levels in your blood. You may have heard *eat leafy green calcium-rich vegetables loaded with calcium*, foods like Kale, turnips, spinach, and collard greens. Other great sources of calcium are cheeses, yogurt, milk and sardines, to name a few. Many people take supplements with calcium and Vitamin D added.

Consuming an unhealthy diet, like the *Standard American Diet*, fast food, junk food, greasy foods, an over abundance of sweets, carbonated beverages, etc. sets up a chemical nightmare of acidity within your body. Additionally, lack of proper calcium levels in your blood can cause *osteoporosis* and a mixed bag of other health problems like those listed above. Is it any wonder so many American's have *acid indigestion, acid reflux disease,* and *peptic ulcers* (located on the duodenum or stomach), etc?

A high acid state destroys your body and a high acid state robs your bones of calcium.

Other contributing factors causing an over abundance of acid in your body is:

- Alcoholic Beverages (wine not included)
- Anger
- Anorexia
- Being Over Worked
- Diabetes
- Excess of Physical Exercise
- Fear
- Fluid Loss (diarrhea, vomiting)
- Kidney Disease
- Over Eating and Over Indulging
- Prescription Drug Use
- Stress
- Tobacco and Tobacco Products
- Toxic Build Up

What are the long-term effects of too much acid in your system?

First, an oversupply of acid leads to depression of a vital system we discussed in the first chapter. That system is the CNS (Central Nervous System), which makes it difficult for you to think clearly, spontaneously, or make decisions quickly. What is the worst case scenario? You can go into a coma and die.

Not to panic. There is a test you can administered to obtain your pH level. You can use a *pH balance test paper*. This paper will give you the acidity or alkalinity values within your body gathered either from your urine or your saliva.

Who sells pH balance test paper? Many health food stores sell this particular test paper. If your health food store does not sell it, just ask for it and I'm sure it's an easy order for them.

Is there a good, better, or best time to test your urine or saliva for pH? It's best to test early in the morning hours. The most accurate and best reliable number is going to be found two hours before you eat or drink anything.

The test is not rocket science. Just slush the existing saliva around in your mouth, spit it in the trash, flush it down the toilet, or swallow it. Work up another good batch, swish it around in your mouth a bit, and then place some of the saliva in your mouth onto the test paper.

If you want to test your urine, just get a clean-catch (the way you do in the lab if you are producing a urine sample and placing it in a clear cup to give to the lab-tech for a urinalysis). Use a throw away cup at home, dip the tip of the test paper into the urine using one-half to three-quarter inch of the test paper, and you'll get an instant reading of your pH balance.

When you get your results, the test scale will read either *logarithmic* or *exponential*. Logarithmic or exponential uses a scale which gives you member values.

Six Chemical Functions Required for Peak Health

Ok, you say. *I've got the results. I have the number value for my pH, now what? What is my next move?*

Depending on your results you can choose to ignore low pH Balance or work to get your pH in balance.

For peak performance and your ultimate goal of good health, it's important to know what is at stake. For you to be in peak shape keep on reading. To be at your peak your body should be able to:

- Detoxify Pollutants & Other Toxic Chemicals
- Detoxify Pollutants from Your Own Waste Products
- Neutralize the Chemical Imbalances Caused by Stress
- Oxygenate Tissues & Cells
- Produce Digestive Enzymes
- Produce Sex Hormones
- Regulate Your Body's Acid/Alkaline Balance

If you get a reading of 6.5 or lower you are in big trouble. Once your pH is out of balance, it may take as long as six months to a full year to get it back in balance. At such times, it is a good idea to use calcium supplements and alter your lifestyle.

First, buy a good supply of calcium supplements, which will quickly start working to balance pH and alkalize your body. One of the best supplements is Coral Calcium. It acts fast inside your body.

Second, take in lots of sunlight in the morning and afternoon. You don't want it to be too hot. Think of sunlight as your magic genie in a jar. Don't stay out in the sun until you turn to toast, but do get 2-3 hours of exposures. Why direct sunlight?

Sunlight acts as a major player in photosynthesis of Vitamin D and INSP-3 in your skin. Once this happens, your body raises the pH of its fluids. Most people don't think about their pituitary gland and hypothalamus needing unfiltered sunlight, but they do. Unfiltered sunlight helps your body know when to eat, sleep, whether to heat up or cool down, signals sexual desires, regulates hormones, and balances water within your body.

Where do you begin? The best place to begin working on your pH balance is by changing your diet; ensuring you eat more foods rich in alkalizing properties and less in acidifying properties. Please review the list below for healthy, wholesome foods to get you started right away.

Foods rich in alkaline:

- Alfalfa
- Apples
- Avocados
- Cherries
- Coconut (fresh)
- Corn
- Dates
- Figs
- Fresh Fruits
- Grapefruit
- Honey
- Horseradish
- Lemons
- Lima Beans
- Maple Syrup
- Molasses
- Mushrooms
- Raisins

- Raspberries
- Soy Sauce
- Sprouts
- Strawberries
- Vinegar
- Watercress
- Vegetables:
- Kudzo
- Onions
- Potatoes
- Rutabagas

Have you heard people say chew your food fifty times? There is an added bonus for chewing your food a long time. The plus is: enzymes in saliva work to reduce acid.

Another perpetrator is red meat. You'll notice a triple cheese burger weighing in at 1 ¼ pounds was not on the list. Therefore, avoid eating too much red meat. Limit your red meat consumption per week to twenty ounces or less. Also limit the amount of sweet, carbonated beverages you consume. Why the caution?

Both red meat and carbonated beverages are loaded with phosphates. Every time you drink a 32-ounce soda you are contributing to a chemical discharge inside your body that is busily at work robbing you of mineral nutrients. Some folks drink several over-sized sodas each day. And the #1 mineral robbed from your body is, you guessed it –calcium.

Good meat choices are chicken and fish; both low in phosphates.

Of course, eat lots of salad greens and rich green veggies. Most people digest salads and vegetables well, while others do not. Make sure you know if you digest these foods well.

You may want to consider juicing. Loading up on nutritiously delicious fruits and vegetables is a quick way to make a major lifestyle change that will change your body pH balance fast. Discover huge packages of cut up kale in the produce section of your grocer or superstore; add carrots, celery, cucumbers, bananas, grapes, oranges, honey, etc. Try to always go with or-ganic fruits and vegetables.

Why go organic? Petroleum-based fertilizers used on crops, along with harmful pesticides kill off 10-20 percent of foods nutritional value. These petroleum-based fertilizers and chemicals kill organisms in the soil which are most beneficial to sound nutrition.

Do you get sick a lot, get indigestion too much, feel out-of-sorts, or feel drained of energy? You could be suffering from *toxic overload*. Did you know when your body is not in pH balance the acid accumulating in your body reduces your body's ability to detox harmful toxins from your body? Again, enter the advantages of adding calcium supplements and adding the calcium housed in leafy green vegetables to your diet.

Six Chemical Functions Required for Peak Performance

Ok, let's say you are doing exactly what you should be doing to put your body in its best pH balance. What are the benefits you can expect to receive from your hard work? You should:

- Get rid of toxins, pollutants, and harmful chemicals, and your own waste
- Neutralize chemical imbalances caused by stress
- Oxygenate tissues and cells
- Produce sex hormones
- Regularly produce digestive enzymes
- Regulate your body's acidalkaline balance

The more in pH balance you are the more functions you'll discover operating to keep you in the peak performance zone.

Eight Traits Necessary to
Maintain Peak Performance

When pH balance is working within your body, chemical functions work to support eight traits which are necessary for you to maintain peak performance. They are:

- Calm, effective, able to handle stress

- Energetic, vitality and physical stamina

- Good camaraderie with others

- Mental alertness, clarity and acuity

- Positive attitude, optimism and goal setting

- Rapid recovery from injury, illness or over exertion

- Resistance to illness

- Spoton in pursuing goals, determined and persistent

Think clearly and analytically and be on your game when your pH is in balance.

Benefits of Electro Physical Medicine
in Restoring pH Balance

We've covered how important it is for your body to self-regulate itself. We've discussed how certain medicines and foods interfere with your body's ability to self-regulate itself. Sometimes we misinterpret our body's natural ability to stay in harmony. Most of us do not consider, nor do we regard the benefits of using electro physical medicine to restore proper pH balance. Perhaps you haven't taken this amazing technological miracle into consideration until now.

The whole genius of this technology lays in the working mechanisms which uses *electrical stimulation* to motivate the skin to do what it should do naturally –heal itself.

Remember, we said your body is a perfectly organized machine designed to heal itself? When your body is out of sync, it cannot do the job it was created to do. Your body has specific active points that respond to minutely sensitive external action. Prick your finger with a needle and you are going to react. Think of this analogy in understanding the organs in your body which are fine-tuned to send data 24/7 about the condition and disorders within your body to your skin. The awesome ability of your body to send messengers through your cells to the skin about failures within your body affecting organs is amazing.

Just as you respond to pricking or cutting your finger with a sharp object, your body is a working system exposed to outside influences affecting it. Your body is like an information highway constantly exchanging data, energy, and conditions of its internal energy with its environment. Think of it as a giant motherboard for all your working parts.

Electro Physical Medicine uses a machine to restore your body's pH balance. In doing so, it restores your organ functions to normal, and stimulates your immune system to protect your body. It does this magnificent feat by transmitting electrical signals through your skin to the internal environment of your body. The input signals are tiny, but your brain has an incredible ability to take the smallest of electrical stimulation and amplify signals. As the reticular formation in your brain magnifies signals put out by this machine, it provides sensations that triggers your immune system to setup your body's defense mechanisms to protect your body and restore it to perfection.

What conditions can you hope to see improvement in when using Electro Physical Medicine? You can expect changes in:

- Acute Diseases
- Chronic Diseases
- Contusions
- Depression
- Headaches
- Impotence Stress Related
- Improve Blood Circulation

- Improvement in Osteoporosis

- Increased Oxygen Supply

- Inflammation

- Muscle Spasms

- Nervous Exhaustion

- Nervous Exhaustion

- Neurological Pain

- Overstrain of Muscles

Now that we know what Electro Physical Medicine can do, let us take a closer look at *SCENAR and Comsodic Technology.*

SCENAR and Comsodic Technology

We live in a world that is constantly changing. Each year new technologies replace old, worn out outdated ones. For example, look at computers and the technological advances made in them in the last twenty-five years. Look at 3D printing and the revolutionary implications of this groundbreaking technology. Both of these innovations and more we've witnessed in our lifetimes. When you or I do not take advantage of new technologies for the betterment of our lives—we first lose, our loved ones are at a loss, family and friends lose, our coworkers lose, our community loses, the organizations and groups we interact with lose, and our significant others and spouse's lose.

If you are like millions and millions of folks on the globe and you embrace innovation, bravo for you. You possess a progressive spirit that recognizes change for the betterment of all humankind is a good thing.

In the previous few pages we covered the triumph technology of using a machine to stimulate the nerve impulses in the body to communicate with the brain through the cellular level of the skin to make positive changes in your body's internal environment. Now, we are going to go one step further and offer further explanation to decipher what *SCENAR and Comsodic Technology* is and how it benefits you and your overall health.

To begin, S-C-E-N-A-R stands for Self Controlled Energetic Neuro-Adaptive-Receptor; now you know why they abbreviated it. Say that ten times with a twist of lemon.

The invention of SCENAR is as impressive as its long name. Back in the day, Alexander Karasev of Russia designed a device as an *informational analogue of a living system*. He actually invented this living system to travel with Russian astronauts to outer space so they could self-administer the healing effects of a hand-held electrical tool to relieve pain while on their voyage. Though the device was never used, it remains one of the more notable inventions of the Twentieth Century. Some have called the SCENAR an *analogue of a living system* and a *health companion for life*. You may call it astonishing when you see how fast, safe and effective it works at assisting living systems to heal themselves.

When we began this chapter, we concentrated on *Electro Physical Medicine*. SCENAR is the machine that makes Electro Physical Medicine possible.

Think of SCENAR as an "ideal electrotherapy" device capable of transmitting signals through your skin, to your brain, and think of this machine as being an "energetic extension" that goes beyond electromagnetism and travels to the heart of your pain.

Some practitioners call *S*CENAR therapy *art*, others refer to it as *science*. I'm sure when the computer was first invented people referred to it as the *Whatchamacallit* or *Whatsit*, etc.

The most important observation, however is, does it work? The answer to this question is a resounding, *yes*. Many users report relief from pain, injuries and illnesses, both chronic conditions and newly acquired conditions. Some of the testimonials may be due to the increases noted in cell rejuvenation by, reportedly, 150%; which alone accelerated the healing process.

For most of us quality of life is paramount. If you're hurting, you usually feel like you are hurting all over. What is so unique about this electronic device is its seemingly uncanny way of automatically analyzing your pain, measuring it, assessing it, then in fractions of a second determining your cell's needs and then automatically delivering a speedy solution. Ask yourself:

- Do you want degenerative tissues to awaken and start regeneration?

- Do you need fast and powerful pain relief?

- Do you need to reduce swelling and inflammation?

- Do you need to improve or begin to restore nerve conductivity and nerve functioning?

- Do you need your body to communicate with itself and start releasing the assistance of healing chemicals?

- Is speeding up your body's ability to recover from traumatic injury important to you?

- Is reversing the signs of aging on your bucket-list?

- Do you want the energy, vitality, and overall health you enjoyed in your youth?

- If you are wondering why your get-up-and-go has got-up-and-gone, ask yourself:

- Would you like to improve the capacity you have for physical endurance?

- Is mental focus important to you?

- What if you could supercharge your productivity, would this be an area you'd like to improve?

- Are flexibility, suppleness and plasticity important to you?

- Do you have a positive outlook on life and would you like to strengthen it?

- Could you use a jump-start on your physical, mental, emotional, and social sense?

- Is making stress a thing of the past a goal you'd like to entertain?

- Is improving your body's ability to heal itself important to you?

- Is hormonal balance an area you'd like to see improvement in?

- Could you use an improvement in your digestion?

- Do you feel you are heart healthy and you have little or no plaque in your arteries?

- Are you stiff, joins showing the strains of worn out cartilages, and is your bone structure not what it used to be?

- Is your memory sharp, or do consistency in thoughts seem to evade you?

- If a good, sound night's sleep were within your grasp, would you reach out and take it?

- If renewed energy is important to you, and you are sick and tired of feeling exhausted and drained, wouldn't you change if you could?

The truth is people just like you are enjoying the new revolutionary treatment that is making effective change in all areas of their body. People are seeing trained techs visit their home or office for *Electro Physical Medicine* applications. Millions are witnessing many benefits each and every time through the use of SCENAR and COSMODIC treatments. In the age of a healthcare system that oftentimes seems on the backburner for many of us, it is refreshing to know a large number of communities across the globe are getting inline to experience the healing effects of *Electro Physical Medicine*. Additionally, many in the medical community are enhancing their practice by adding one or more machines to their professional clinics and adding trained personnel to administer to their patients.

As we said in the beginning of this chapter, "A body in perfect balance is like a fine oiled and fine tuned working machine. Your body's pH balance is essential to your good health. Maintaining your body's proper pH balance is vital to your health in avoiding chronic and degenerative diseases…" SCENAR & COSMODIC therapy gives your body maximum results to heal.

In the next chapter, we are going to explore further and dive deeply into *Pulsed Electro Magnetic Field Therapy*.

CHAPTER **3**

Pulsed Electro Magnetic Field Therapy

You are probably most familiar with *electrothera-py*, not to be confused with *electroconvulsive therapy* or *electroshock therapy*. *Pulsed Electro Magnetic Field Therapy* uses regulated, pulsating stimulation enhanced by **electromagnetic energy**. When you apply pulsation and stimulation with the added benefit of an electrical devise, you specifically **target electric current to speed wound healing**.

This technology has been applied to many alternative medical devices used over the years. It has aided in the effective treatment of bone healing.

Electrical Muscle Stimulation

Pulsed Electro Magnetic Field Therapy has proven through research to speed up the healing of wounds. A study performed in 2000 by the *Dutch Medical Council* discovered that regardless of its wide use, it did not have sufficient evidence to prove the benefits. However, what a difference ten years makes. Today, the use of **electrotherapy is breaking new ground as it helps patients rehabilitate.** The APTA (American Physical Therapy Association) endorses the use of electrotherapy for pain management, noting improvements in range-of-motion exercises enabling patients to move more freely.

An added bonus to patients using Pulsed Electro Magnetic Field Therapy is that the electrical stimulation retards and prevents muscle atrophy and it also has a restorative affect. Pulsed Electro Magnetic Field Therapy also:

- Restored Muscle Mass

- Strengthened Muscles

- Demonstrated Destruction of Cancer Tumors up to 60% (1985 journal on Cancer Research)

- Reported 98% shrinkage of tumors in animal subjects (same study as above)

- Aids in pain management

- Improved range-of-motion, joint movement
- Aids in the treatment of neuromuscular dysfunction

Who wouldn't want improvement of strength, or improvement of motor control, or to retard muscles from wasting away (atrophy), or who would not want to improve local blood flow?

The medical profession today relies too heavily on pain medication administered through prescription drug therapy. Often ignoring the benefits short-term and long-term gained from using Pulsed Electro Magnetic Field Therapy.

Many patients are over-medicated due to needing more drug therapy to counteract an original prescribed drug. One man, reportedly, was taken sixteen medications. When opting for a second opinion, he discovered he only needed two.

Why does this oversight continue to occur within the medical community?

The man above, Dan, said the second doctor he visited told him, *you are taking the 3ʳᵈ medication to prevent upset stomach and diarrhea, which is a bad side-effect of that particular drug. You are taking the 4ᵗʰ medication to counter the side-effects of headache and nausea, a side-effect of drug #3, so on* and so on and weary so on…

Today, more than ever before, it pays to be health-smart and question your physician about what he or she is prescribing that is entering your body. A middle-age woman named Sara (not her real name for confidentiality purposes), tells her story.

I didn't feel real sick, but I did feel overly tired. I went to the ER and was told my blood-work came back questionable, and just for a precautionary measure, I'd be admitted to the hospital for overnight and for further evaluation.

A few hours later, while in my hospital room, a nurse entered my room holding a medication in the form of a needle; as she was telling me how worn out and tired she was from working a 12-hour shift, and agreeing to stay two additional hours due to low-staffing levels, I interrupted her ramblings and asked her, "Is that shot for me?" She responded, "Yes it is Sweety; a shot to ease your pain."

I protested, "I'm not in pain. What is in that syringe?"

She replied, "Morphine."

Shocked, I nearly screamed out, "Do you see the red band on my arm? I'm allergic to morphine. Do you want to kill me?"

As disbelieving as this may sound, it is a true account of a hospital nightmare. Unfortunately, it is much too real. Sara explained to her daughter later, "If you hadn't warned me to always ask what medications medical staff was administering to me, I would have never asked. I always trusted my doctor and medical staff and never asked any questions fearing I'd offend someone. Boy, am I glad you gave me that advice.

IF you are much like Sara and have never asked a lot of questions, and perhaps trusted too much in medical staff caring for you, isn't it time you started asking many questions about the care you are given and the medications you're prescribed?

Why do some people seem to stay sick all the time, while others seemingly enjoy good health? Is it the luck of the draw? It's your turn on the evolutionary-scale to get sick, or is it an area you can control yourself?

A human being is the top of the evolutionary tree of the organic world, noted Dr. Yuri Gorfinkel, 1998:

It possesses the most perfect *structure* and performs the most sophisticated *functions*. And since the human body is perfect by design, the mechanisms of self-regulation of this body should also be perfect.

We were not designed by nature to get sick. Foreign invaders (germs) are supposed to be dealt with immediately. Our body is hypothetically supposed to notice little to no change in our internal environment as the invaders are eradicated by the body's defense mechanism.

What's going on IF we continually get sick?

We Are Our Own Worst Enemy

A huge contributing factor is us. We are in essence our own worst enemy. Though we've continued to evolve as a people, though we've continued to accomplish great feats in scientific discoveries, we forgot how to use self-regulation. On an ongoing basis, we wreck havoc with different forms of treatment, again, self-regulation. We miss the signals the body sends out. We miss the internal clues given to us by our body. We are so scared of dying, we stress out over living.

You've heard the expression, *Life is for the living*. You are not designed to suffer. You're made to enjoy life and all its pleasures and rewards. The more you reap in positive emotions and good health, the fuller your life is. The bonus is: A healthier you.

Ok, you say, *now you've got my attention. What can I do to make me happier and healthier?*

Get Rid of Your Physical Suffering

IS it possible to get rid of physical suffering? What if I shared this with you? You can ease your pain the first time you experience a SCENAR session, or Pulsed Electro Magnetic Field Therapy. Would eliminating pain give you a greater chance to face the world each day more optimistic and more positive about your life and your future?

Of course it would make a huge difference in the quality and prospects for longevity in your life.

As we said earlier in this chapter, your body has its own detection system to ward off disease so you are able to function and carry on with your daily routine.

The best news yet, your body's amazing equipment has the ability to act like a sonar device and diagnose what's going on internally. In *Pulsed Electro Magnetic Field Therapy* it really doesn't matter what your diagnosis is or how long you've suffered from a particular disease. What matters is how you feel and how you articulate to others about your pain level.

As you progress in using this therapy, you'll notice changes in the way you feel the first sessions and every session thereafter. Since you body carries out the repair of its functions, you'll notice the restorative processes affecting the internal mechanics of your body right away.

Think of your body as an entire system. No one part is independent without the others. Thinking of your body as *movable parts divided* (if you will), is improper.

To clarify this point, the medical profession fails greatly when a practitioner, for instance, prescribes a conventional medicine that treats one symptom at the expense of other healthy body parts. Sure, you may feel better and the body part the drug was supposed to make feel better does feel better. But if the drug prescribed destroys your liver in the long run, what have you really benefited? Isn't that like playing *Russian Roulette*?

Using Pulsed Electro Magnetic Field Therapy

When you're using Pulsed Electro Magnetic Field Therapy, you are in control. You turn it on, or have a technician administer therapy to you, and you feel results. It is that simple.

If you are suffering from debilitating illnesses or diseases, PEMFT, also aids in tissue repair by enhancing microcirculation and protein synthesis to heal damaged tissue. It also restores the integrity of the connective and dermal tissues.

If you have witnessed edema on yourself or on another person suffering from edema, you know how heart-wrenching torn tissue looks, and you may know how it feels. Edema can accumulate in tissues, especially in the lower legs and extremities until it literally splits the skin apart. Skin open to the environment can usher in bacteria and leave the affected person open to life-threatening infections.

Treatment with PEMFT accelerates the absorption rate, lessening the painful effects of edema. Treatment also affects blood vessel permeability, increases mobility proteins, blood cells and lymphatic flow, peripheral blood flow, induces arterial, venous and lymphatic flow.

Further Benefits of Electro Magnetic Field Therapy

IF you've always believed the only kind of treatment for illness or injury was conventional medicine administered by a conventional medical person, then welcome to the 21st Century. PEMFT (Pulsed Electro Magnetic Field Therapy) transmits electrical signals through your skin; though electrical signals are minute, the reticular formation in your brain amplifies the signals, resulting in stimulating your defense mechanisms within your body. PEMFT can:

- Normalize Organ Functions
- Stimulate Immune Systems

- Stimulate Other Protective Mechanisms within the Body
- Aids in the delivery of pharmacological medication
- Aids in Urine and fecal incontinency, affecting the pelvic floor, works to reduce pelvic pain and build stronger musculature in this area
- Give positive hope that may lead to complete continence
- Asserts to Control the Systems of the Human Body
- Makes it Possible to Treat Various Diseases & Conditions with Your Body

Your body and Pulsed Electro Magnetic Field Therapy work together, much akin to the electric signals generated by your own biological processes. The similarity between the two systems, allows both systems to work together. This breakthrough technology creates a balance of interaction between the device and your biological processes. The electrical impulses are tiny, but the reticular formation within your brain enables the signals to amplify; thus stimulating the defense mechanisms within your body.

What You Can Expect From Pulsed Electro Magnetic Field Therapy

In addition to the benefits we've already covered, you can also expect Pulsed Electro Magnetic Field Therapy to work with your body to heal:

- Acute Diseases

- Chronic Diseases

Both disorders caused by chaos in some of our body organs which cause them to malfunction.

Help You Help Yourself

There are other avenues you can take to help you help yourself. Among these are:

- Deep breathing

- Inhale through your nose

- Exhale through your mouth

- Repeat 1020 times

- Pace yourself

The above exercises will help you control the acidity within your body which contributes to degeneration. This degeneration affects your entire body system.

You, your loved ones, and people you've never met benefit daily from Pulsed Electro Magnetic Field Therapy. Trained technicians span the globe. Preventive measures aid in healing, and help your body heal faster. PEMFT works with your body to heal itself. Get relief from:

- Muscle Spasms
- Prevent & Retard Disused Muscles, stop atrophy
- Increase Blood Flow
- Increase Blood Circulation
- Rehabilitate Muscles
- Train Muscles with Electrical Muscle stimulation
- Maintain Range-of-Motion
- Increase Movement
- Manage Chronic Pain
- Mange Post-Traumatic Acute Pain
- Manage Post-Surgical Acute Pain
- Stimulate Post-Surgical Muscles to Prevent Venous Thrombosis
- Speed Wound Healing
- Speed Medication Delivery

Reduce the pain, speed the healing process, while allowing your body to work as it was designed to work. Keeping your body fine-tuned and receptive to signals it relies on to heal are absolutely paramount in the healing process.

Don't leave the healing of your body to chance. Don't sit around and passively wait for drugs to ease your pain while you hope your body heals itself on its own. Get with a trained professional, and find out firsthand what you need to do to take advantage of this amazing technology.

We've discussed the importance of proper pH Balance throughout this book. In the next chapter, we're going to take a closer look at using specialized ionic water to re-establish the pH Balance in your body.

CHAPTER 4

Using Specialized Ionic Water to Re-Establish pH Balance

You've heard pH Balance a lot, but did you know pH stands for "potential of hydrogen", and that basically it is the concentration of hydrogen ions in a solution?

We mentioned earlier the scale, but let's look at the *potential of hydrogen* as it is measured on a scale of 0.00 to 14.00. We also mentioned earlier, a ranking above 7.00 indicates a substance is alkaline. When we go lower than 7.00, we said it is *acid*.

Armed with this information, we look at pure water and notice it has a pH closer to *neutral* (7.00).

This is a good indication of why your doctor orders lab-work, more specifically "blood-work" because a slight increase or decrease in the whole number may indicate a problem (acidity or alkalinity).

It's important to understand the numbers, before you can fully appreciate the benefits obtained from using specialized ionic water to re-establish pH balance.

It is also equally important to know when acidic and alkaline substances are mixed together, they *neutralize* each other. We talked earlier about the trillions of cells in our bodies; each a fluid-filled assembly containing a lot of alkaline substances. Minerals like:

- Bicarbonate
- Calcium
- Magnesium
- Oxygen
- Potassium
- Sodium

When all these minerals are combined within the cell they contribute to a small alkaline intracellular pH (above 7.00). Therefore, keep in mind; the cells are surrounded by fluids containing alkaline minerals.

Water Ionizer Systems

Technology has come a long way since your great-grandmother turned on a tap to fetch a glass of water. Today, smart tech-savvy devices use simple water from your faucet, pass it through a filtration and electrolysis, and *Walla* –alkaline water appears; which has amazing health benefits. Millions of units each year find their way into kitchens across the globe.

Here's how it works.

The countertop devise is a tad taller than a big the-saurus (standing tall), fits neatly on your countertop. Other devices connect to the water source (under the sink models). Both perform electrolysis of the water as it passes through the internal chambers of the machine. This process works on the principle that positive (+) ions attract to negative (-) ions. What remains is water with an excess of electrons. This is a good thing, be-cause this process raises the pH levels in the water to between 9 and 11. Your water, fully transformed after it passes from the electrolysis chamber is ready to use for drinking or cooking.

The electrolysis process removes:

- Chlorine
- Impurities
- Odors
- What can you do with alkaline water? You can:
- Clean Fruit & Veggies
- Sanitize Cutting Boards
- Sanitize Knives, Forks, Spoons & Other Utensils

- Use as a Sterile Water to Clean Wounds
- Use for Skincare
- Wash Your Hands

Hydrating Effects of Alkaline Water

The alkaline water reduces by 50%; which allows for rapid absorption by your body. This increases the hydrating effects of the water, and also influences your body's ability to carry its negative ions and alkalinizing effects to every cell and tissue in your body.

Why is this process important to you and to you maintaining proper pH balance in your body? Water treated in this way, not only surpasses its ability to slowly raise your pH within your cells, but it raises the pH of each cell in your body, it raises the pH in your tissues, and it neutralizes acids in your body. How does it do this?

As the tap water goes through electrolysis, it gains a large number of free electrons; it is then able to give these electrons to active oxygen radicals within your body.

Your Healthy GI Track Depends on pH Balance

Why focus on pH balance? The metabolic and enzymatic reactions in your body, in my body, in all bodies function in smooth working order in an alkaline environment. To include:

- Digestion

- Energy Production

- Immunity

- Repairing your body

Keeping your body in proper pH balance allows all those trillions of cells the oxygen they require to function to their fullest. Keep in mind, when your body is in pH balance you feel good, energized, and all the while glucose and vital nutrients continually breakdown to convert to adenosine triphosphate. Your Healthy GI Track Depends on pH Balance.

Key: Rich Alkaline Environment

Benefits of Healthy Digestive-Enzymes

Help improve your overall productivity by knowing and implementing healthy digestive-enzyme production. You'll enjoy:

- Added Physical Vitality

- Enhanced Acuity

- Faster recovery from injuries

- Increased Mental Clarity

- Increased Stamina

- More at ease with coworkers, family and friends

- Quicker recovery from illnesses

Bounce back from inflammations:

- Allergies
- Athletic Injuries
- Bronchitis
- Common Colds
- Dental Procedures
- Flu
- Minor Surgery
- Repetitive-stress Injuries
- Sinusitis

Simple, daily changes add up to big health benefits. You will optimize digestion, while improving absorption of nutrients and your body will be better able to tolerate medications, thus increasing the effectiveness of medicines you must take.

Who does not want to lower the risk of inflammatory diseases? The first disease that readily comes to mind is the debilitating effects of rheumatoid arthritis, or the aggravating effects of colitis, and:

- Endometriosis
- Prostatitis
- Thyroiditis

Other health benefits:

- Accelerates healing from existing heart disease
- Accelerates healing from stroke
- Accelerates healing of blood clots
- Decreases the risk of heart disease
- Enhances therapy for the treatment of cancer

IF you feel you do not have good digestive-enzyme production, perhaps you should ask yourself why.

Alkalizing Products

To restore your acid/alkaline balance, several alkalizing products are available. The fastest way to stay in balance if you're in trouble is to add adequate intake in your diet of:

- Calcium
- Magnesium
- Mineral Supplements
- Potassium

Those listed and using alkalinizing therapies like Pulsed Electro Magnetic Field Therapy (key here: magnetic field) are quick remedies. Also, it's a good idea to exercise regularly, a moderate aerobic exercise is best. Some folks head to a favorite, peaceful spot to relieve stress where they can meditate and reflect, while others practice deep breathing, relaxation techniques and yoga.

It's best to stay aware of practices that work to destroy your pH balance. It's even better to know what to do when you realize you're in trouble.

- Aspirin (acidforming drugs)
- Becoming better accustomed to adding acidic minerals, phosphorus, sulfur to your daily regimen

High-alkaline Producers:

- Add a shot of cider vinegar to your day
- Include more acidic, nutrient-rich foods in your diet
- Supplements like hydrochloric acid
- Vitamin C

Of course each one actively benefits the other, but acid-enhancing habits like fast-paced exercise or physically challenging activities contributes to getting your pH out of balance, as does an overly active lifestyle.

Relaxation of Injured Tissue (Ion Gates)

No, we are not talking about iron gates, but *ion gates*. Ion Gates have an important role when it comes regulating the flow of proteins in and out of the cells. See the Role of Ion Gates below:

The ion gates are protein channels that regulate ion flow into and out of the cell. There are three gates that are associated with the action potential: m, h, and n. The m and h gates control sodium flow, while the n gate controls potassium flow. In the resting phase of the action potential, the m gate is closed, while the h gate is open. Therefore, sodium is neither leaving or entering the cell. The n gate is also closed, so potassium can neither leave nor enter the cell. During depolarization, the m gate opens allowing sodium to diffuse down its gradient, while the n gate is still closed. During repolarization, the h gate closes, preventing sodium from coming into the cell. The n gate is open during this phase so potassium moves out. In the undershoot phase, the m gate closes, the h gate stays closed, and the n gate stays open. Finally, the h gate opens, the n gate closes and resting state is once again achieved. This is illustrated in the figure below.

(A) = Resting State
(B) = Depolarization Phase
(C) = Repolarization Phase
(D) = Undershoot

Above information taken directly from:
http://www.shodor.org/Hodgkin/index.html

Ion Gates during Nerve Action Potential

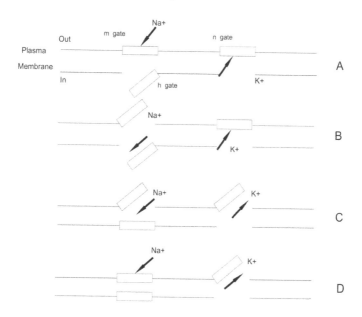

Restoration of Injured Tissue

The medical dictionary defines wound healing as, *a process to restore to a state of soundness to any injury that results in an interruption in the continuity of external surfaces of the body.*

Yet, tissue repair not only takes regeneration and restoration of the injured tissue, it includes taking into account the scarring associated with the injury. Anytime you suffer an injury, your first concern is survival, and your second concern is restoring your body to balance (healing).

Restoration of Function

After injury, if you cannot carry out the functions necessary for you to perform your daily activities of life, be it vocational or recreational, you have a problem. Most of us do not want to rely on loved ones for long. The healing process can take its toll on family members. Your first concern should be restoration of physiological function, a renewal of normal cellular activity.

Using alkalinizing agents to speed healing is on the rise; be it a type of acute injury, traumatic or tissue damaged from a surgical procedure. Any injury to your body causes the damaged tissue to become acidic, oftentimes, overly acidic. This creates extra stress on your buffering capabilities. Why does injured tissue become acidic?

When you or I are injured and the injury results are tissue damage, the injured tissue swells, sometimes hemorrhage follows, and we simultaneously feel other physical changes taken place within our body. For one, we'll feel the impaired oxygenation to the affected tissue/s. Then the damage intensifies when blood flow to the area diminishes, and waste products begin accumulating, which intensifies acidity. Then toss in metabolic activities on steroids, protein synthesis, and you have the perfect storm (so to speak). Now, you have a body in healing overdrive, as your body's healing processes arm itself to repair the damage.

Below is the best advice from experts:

If you are overly acidic and tend to recover slowly from injuries, begin an alkalinizing program immediately following an acute injury. This should be done whether the injury is incurred taking part in strenuous physical activity or is due to trauma or surgery, because injuries are always accompanied by inflammation…

A healthy alkaline balance puts you way ahead of the game. Knowing how important proper pH balance is in achieving good health gives you an assurance of speed in recovery from injury, illnesses, over exertion, and strengthens your body's resolve to battle illnesses that may come your way.

Recharging the System

You've heard the saying, *you've come a long way, baby*. Recharging your system is an ongoing process. Many of us fail to realize fully the importance in keeping the liver in maximum working order. The liver continually detoxifies pollutants you ingest or absorb from your immediate environment, from your work environment, and from your community. We'll touch briefly on some steps you can take to reestablish your liver's ability to detoxify.

When you first begin detoxing to cleanse your liver, be aware you may experience fatigue, headaches, flu-like symptoms, etc. so you want to start slow.

The first thing you'll want to do is cleanse your colon. Go with a colon cleansing agent that works best for you. One good colon cleanse on the market is *Trifgol*.

Note: The author and its publishers do not make monetary gain from mentioning *Trifgol*, nor do we attest to its effectiveness.

Once you cleanse your colon, you may want to follow with 2-3 days of juicing. There are many good juicing books in the marketplace with recipes, many containing sound advice on adapting a clean, wholesome lifestyle.

You'll want to consider eating a mostly vegetarian diet; raw foods like salads, variety of greens, fresh veggies, whole grains, nuts and legumes. Go easy on animal proteins; depend on fish and eggs instead. Watch out for butter, solid shortenings, lard, and opt instead for vegetable oils. For a list of vegetarian diets, and to distinguish from Vegan, Lactovegetarian, and ovo-vegetarian dies, check out his helpful link: http://www.webmd.com/food-recipes/guide/vegetarian-and-vegan-diet

You'll hear many people swearing by a *good ole commonsense fast*, but this book does not recommend fasting. Those committing to a true fast may only consume water, diluted, weak soups, juices, chicken or beef broths, herbal teas, etc for 3, 5, and 7 days. Fasting may get you into trouble. If you must take this route (excuse the expression), in cleansing your colon, we recommend you consult a physician and be under his or her care prior to you embarking on a fasting routine.

You'll also want to take a multi vitamin-mineral supplement to maintain basic Detox nutrients. Follow this helpful link for more information. http://www.thorne.com/Products/Detoxification/prd~VMD.jsp

Recharging the System Through pH Balance

Throughout this book, we've given you many tools you can use to recharge your system through pH balance. Do:

- Follow an alkaline diet

Work to restore alkaline mineral reserves in your cells, tissues and bones

- Check out vitamin-mineral supplements
- Eat wholesome foods to ensure proper colon cleansing
- Opt for foods that are more alkaline
- Stay away from acid-forming foods
- Stay away from high acidic foods

- Talk with your physician about what's best for you

- Vary foods in your diet to keep you on track

Perhaps in the history of the human race we didn't need to worry ourselves about the decline in minerals and other nutrients in our diets, but as humans evolved and transitioned from hunter/gathers to farming, and further discovered spices, coupled with a mixed-bag of processed foods, unfortunately, our body's changed too. Adapting to change is often difficult, but you have many of the tools you need to get you on your way to pH balance.

This book, by no means contains all the information available on restoring your body's proper pH balance. We encourage you to read other books on the subject, stay involved in maintaining your pH balance once you have yours under control, and always stay proactive when it comes to your health.

Bonus: Interactive Checklist Discover Why Lifestyle & Environment Affect pH Balance

Take a look at the checklist below, get a pen or pencil and prepare to take the challenge to discover for yourself why your lifestyle and environment may be affecting your health.

Place a checkmark beside the statement that best describes you.

	I drink alcohol excessively.
	I feel out of sorts on a diet consisting mostly of high fats, animal proteins and high sugar content.
	I often feel restricted in my capacity to eat a wide assortment of foods; both in a personal, business and social settings.

	Though I feel I eat a proper amount of food to maintain my health, I fail to have enough energy to carry out simple, daily routines.
	Even small injuries often take much longer to heal than expected.
	Each day after heavy lifting, exercise, or walking, I feel overly stiff, and suffer from soreness in my muscles.
	Some days, it seems whether I'm having fun or working, I tire easily.
	Traveling, even short distances, leaves me exhausted and overly fatigued.
	Oftentimes I experience difficulty thinking straight, and my response time is off.
	I think indigestion is part of the aging process.
	My stomach holds an excessive amount of fluid. I often feel bloated, and suffer from discomfort, especially after eating.
	I take a lot of antacids to feel better.
	For no reason at all, I suffer sudden intestinal cramps after eating that leave me incapable of carrying out simple tasks.
	If I were a hydrogen balloon I'd float above my misery, as I have bouts of flatulence after meals.
	When I have a bowel-movement, I cannot help noticing the stool in the toilet appears undigested, lumpy and greasy.

	I would make a bad baseball player, as I'd have trouble sliding from base-to-base with the chronic diarrhea I often experience.
	On the flip side, after ingesting certain foods, I have stacks of stool packed like rocks one upon the other, adding to a constipation nightmare.
	When I eat fiery foods, rich foods, or zesty and spicy gourmet foods, I have extreme trouble digestion; equivalent to a 4-alarm fire.
	I'm usually totally exhausted after a meal, and often collapse in my recliner or a soft spot on the couch beside the dog.
	I often experience chronic pancreatitis.
	I experience ulcerative colitis.
	I have a long bout with irritable bowel syndrome.
	I have notable history of Crohn's disease (inflammatory bowel disease, affecting the gastrointestinal tract).
	I have had gallstone surgery in the past.
	I'd feel better if rheumatoid arthritis wasn't a daily concern.
	My medical history shows a history of vasculitis.
	I have endometriosis.
	I have food allergies.
	I have environmental allergies.

Okay, before you feel completely deflated from the over-abundance of checkmarks, take a deep breath and relax. Sometimes a cold, hard look at the facts is enough to jolt you into action. It is good to have an understanding of the necessity for you to get your digestive-enzyme production in check. The good news is, your good health is in your hands, and knowledge empowers us to make necessary, positive changes.

Read over the information in this book, review the information again, and prepare yourself to make the lifestyle changes to improve your health by getting your pH balance in order. You are never too young or too old to make constructive changes for the betterment of your health.

Conclusion

As they say in sports, *Game On!* You are way ahead of the game when you consider the many advantages derived from keeping your body's pH balance. You deserve:

- An Optimistic Attitude

- Keeping to task and persevering until you reach your goals

- Mental Accuracy

- Mental Clarity

- Physical Stamina to do the things you want to accomplish

- Physical Vitality

- Quick recovery from exertion, illness and injuries

- Resistance from Illnesses

- Setting goals you can keep

- Stress-free Lifestyle

You and you alone are ultimately in charge of your health. Whether you choose to take care of yourself, or you choose to ignore good, sound advice, and continue on a collision course sure to end in disaster is completely up to you, but don't you owe it to yourself and your loved ones to do everything in your power to stay healthy, reach peak performance; be it in your career, your community, or your family?

References

Webliography
http://scenar.biz/what-is-scenar.html

http://www.scenar-therapy.com/therapy

http://www.shodor.org/Hodgkin/index.html

Bibliography
David, S. L; Absolom, D. R., Smith, C. R., Gams, J., and Herbert, M. A., *Effect of low level direct current on in vivo tumor growth in hamsters.* Cancer Research, 1985.

Gardner SE, Frantz RA, Schmidt FL (1999), *Effect of Electrical stimulation on Chronic Wound Healing: A Meta-Analysis.*

Humphrey, C.E.; Seal, E.H., *Biophysical approach toward tumor regression in mice*, Science, 1959.

Institute of Electrical and Electronics Engineers, *The IEEE Standard Dictionary of Electrical and Electronics Terms*, 6th Ed. New York, NY, Institute of Electrical and Electronics Engineers, 1997.

Kulsh, J., *Targeting a key enzyme in cell growth: a novel therapy for cancer.* Medical Hypotheses, 1997.

Medicine, An Illustrated History by Albert S. Lyons, M.D., F.A.C.S., Clinical Professor of Surgery, Archivist, and Coordinator of History of Medicine, Mount Sinai School of Medicine and R. Joseph Petrucelli, II, M.D., Assistant Professor of Physiology and Biophysics, Lecturer in Medicine, Mount Sinai School of Medicine, published by Harry N. Abrams, Inc., Publishers, New York, NY., 1978.

Mollon B, da Silva V, Busse JW, Einhorn TA, Bhandari M., *Electrical stimulation for long-bone fracture-healing: a meta-analysis of randomized controlled trials.* J Bone Joint Surg Am, November 2008.

Robinson AJ, Snyder-Mackler, L. *Clinical Electrophysiology: Electrotherapy and Electrophysiologic Testing*, 3rd ed. Baltimore, Lippincott Williams and Wilkins, 2008.

The Chemistry Of Success, Secrets Of Peak
Performance by Susan M. Lark, M.D. and James A.
Richards, M.B.A., Bay Books, San Francisco, CA,
2000.

Notes & Thoughts

Dr. Yuri Gorfinkel, 1998: Considered one of the first
and best SCENAR Specialist and Trainer. Parts of his
speech from the first international SCENAR Training
course held in Bahamas in 1997.

Russian Roulette: *A deadly game using a revolver: a
deadly game in which people take turns firing a revolver loaded with only one bullet at their own heads, after
spinning the cylinder; something dangerous: a dangerous or reckless action or activity.*

Encarta ® World English Dictionary © & (P) 1998-2005
Microsoft Corporation.

CPSIA information can be obtained
at www.ICGtesting.com
Printed in the USA
FFHW011603200919
55110095-60814FF